HOME WORKOUT FOR BEGINNERS

The Very Best Collection of Exercise and Fitness Books

(The Essential Guide to Home Workout)

Kenny Morel

Published by Oliver Leish

Kenny Morel

All Rights Reserved

Home Workout for Beginners: The Very Best Collection of Exercise and Fitness Books (The Essential Guide to Home Workout)

ISBN 978-1-77485-190-6

All rights reserved. No part of this guide may be reproduced in any form without permission in writing from the publisher except in the case of brief quotations embodied in critical articles or reviews.

Legal & Disclaimer

The information contained in this book is not designed to replace or take the place of any form of medicine or professional medical advice. The information in this book has been provided for educational and entertainment purposes only.

The information contained in this book has been compiled from sources deemed reliable, and it is accurate to the best of the Author's knowledge; however, the Author cannot guarantee its accuracy and validity and cannot be held liable for any errors or omissions. Changes are periodically made to this book. You must consult your doctor or get professional medical advice before using any of the suggested remedies, techniques, or information in this book.

Upon using the information contained in this book, you agree to hold harmless the Author from and against any damages, costs, and expenses, including any legal fees potentially resulting from the application of any of the information provided by this guide. This disclaimer applies to any damages or injury caused by the use and application, whether directly or indirectly, of any advice or information presented, whether for breach of contract, tort, negligence, personal injury, criminal intent, or under any other cause of action.

You agree to accept all risks of using the information presented inside this book. You need to consult a professional medical practitioner in order to ensure you are both able and healthy enough to participate in this program.

Table of Contents

INTRODUCTION 1

CHAPTER 1: WEIGHT TRAINING FOR WEIGHT LOSS 5

CHAPTER 2: WHAT IS AEROBICS? 9

CHAPTER 3: HOW TO CREATE YOUR AMAZING HOME GYM
.... 18

CHAPTER 4: BEGINNING 27

CHAPTER 5: SUPERMANS 35

CHAPTER 6: QUESTIONS TO ASK BEFORE YOU START A
FITNESS PROGRAM 46

CHAPTER 7: THE THREE MOST IMPORTANT RULES FOR
BODY TRANSFORMATION 50

CHAPTER 8: BASIC STRETCHING 63

CHAPTER 9: ARMS AND LOVE HANDLES 72

CHAPTER 10: DOING AEROBIC EXERCISE AT HOME: WHAT
ARE THE WONDERS? 78

CHAPTER 11: THE BENEFITS OF STAYING FIT 86

CHAPTER 12: WHY YOU SHOULD BE WORKING OUT 93

CHAPTER 13: 30-DAY WORKOUT CHALLENGE................ 106

CHAPTER 14: BODYWEIGHT EXERCISES FOR EASY WEIGHT LOSS 115

CHAPTER 15: TOP DAILY EXERCISES BENEFITS 131

CHAPTER 16: SIMPLE LOWER ABS WORKOUTS FOR WOMEN AT HOME 145

CONCLUSION.. 152

Introduction

These chapters will show you how to work out at home to build muscle and reduce fat. The whole-body workouts can be done at home with strength and muscle as the focal point.

If you don't exercise regularly or haven't been exercising at all, it takes time to build an athletic body. This book will help you achieve your goal faster than if it were you just running on the treadmill for an hour. This book will help you overcome the mental obstacles to sticking to a workout program. It will help you stay motivated, and it will make it easy to track your progress.

This book is unique because it combines strength with weight loss goals. It offers flexibility and toning advice. It is a result of years of training. You can work out at home, and get all the benefits of a gym without needing to travel or pay high-end membership fees. You can make investments in your equipment at home and keep it for many years. You can do most of the exercises in the book without any equipment, or you can use equipment you have at home.

Body Weight workouts will be presented to you. These are exercises that use your own body weight. They include a series of exercises designed to tone and build muscle. These workouts are simple and can be done without any equipment. You can also use the household items in the next chapters. These exercises are a great way to tone and shape your body. This chapter should be used generously.

A section of the book will address limitations in mobility and modify workouts accordingly. This section will cover how yoga poses can increase mobility and improve form and strength. These poses will improve your flexibility and endurance. This chapter will help you improve your focus and strength training.

You'll learn how to modify your workouts, taking it as far as you can. You are free to be creative and combine the workouts from different chapters to create your own program.

We'll discuss how to use the Barbell and Dumbbell chapters with minimal equipment. You will learn barbell skills that you can use for many different workouts and techniques. This will help you build serious muscle and reduce excess fat.

You will also learn useful tips to keep your interest in the exercise program and how you can maximize your results through smart food choices. You can download a 7-Day Meal Plan to help you plan what to eat throughout the week. You can even find desserts and snacks included to help you stay on track and feel satisfied.

As a guide, we have provided some photos.

There are many books available on this topic, so thank you for choosing this one! We made every effort to make sure it was as useful as possible. Please enjoy!

Chapter 1: Weight training for weight loss

Weight training to lose weight may seem odd at first. This is because weight training is often associated with bulk building. Weight training can be a great way to shed extra weight. It works for both men as well as women.

Your muscles will need more calories if you want to increase muscle mass. Because your muscles need more energy to survive, they will do so. Your body will have fewer calories that can be stored as fat. In short, your muscles will begin to eat away some of your body's fat.

Your results will be improved even if you only reduce your calorie intake a little. To achieve the best results, it is important to change your diet plan in order to eat fewer calories and still lose weight.

It's not an easy balance. Your muscles will shrink if you cut back on calories. Your body won't have enough muscles to combat the excess fat. You are making your body starve if you don't eat enough. This causes your brain to go into survival mode which then tells your body that it needs to store fat. You will experience a slowdown in your metabolism, which will also reduce fat burning.

Weight lifting and metabolic exercise

You must increase your metabolism rate to burn fat. Lifting weights is one way to do this. Your metabolism will continue to be high even after you leave the gym, so you can continue reaping the benefits. Your body requires more oxygen when you gain weight. To meet this increased demand, your metabolism will speed up.

Weight lifting can flex your muscles which aids in weight loss. Muscles can play an important role in increasing your metabolism rate, it has been suggested.

One pound more muscle can help you burn around 20 calories per day.

Weight Training and the Brain's Hypothalamus

Weight training is not the only way to lose fat.

Your heart rate increases when you lift weight. Your heart rate increases and the Leptin hormone in blood is more easily transmitted to the brain's receptor, called the hypothalamus. Your brain then can send the right message to your body about whether you should eat more of less. The hypothalamus will then tell your body to eat less if you are overweight. It can use the stored fat as an energy source.

You should aim to lift moderate weight for best results. You are not trying to be a bodybuilder. It is always better to combine lifting weights and cardio exercises. This will allow you to burn more fat faster.

There are many reasons to lift weight. This will increase your endurance and strengthen your bones. People who are overweight sleep better at night. Researchers have found a link between weight gain, insomnia, and other factors. There are many explanations. The most obvious explanation is that the body repairs and restores itself when it is at rest. If you don't get enough sleep, your body's fat-metabolizing mechanisms won't work as efficiently. Well-rested bodily organs will work better. Lift some weights to improve your sleeping habits.

You will also have more energy to do physical activities if your strength increases. This is why bodybuilders and athletes spend hours at the gym. You will be able to run, cycle, or swim for longer and burn more fat.

You can see that there is a link between weight training, weight loss, and both.

Chapter 2: What is Aerobics?

Aerobics, which literally translates to "with oxygen", is a way to lose weight and improve your health. Aerobics can be done in many different ways and you'll soon notice a difference in your health. Aerobics that are moderately intense for longer periods of times target specific body parts. Aerobics has many benefits, making it a popular exercise choice for health-conscious individuals.

There are two types of exercise: anaerobic and aerobic. They differ because of the way muscles contract and how energy is used within them.

Anaerobic exercises include strength training and weight training. Aerobic exercises can make it impossible for even the most fit bodybuilder to run, swim, or do other aerobic activities. For long periods of time.

Aerobics does not require you to use a lot of energy in a short period. To stimulate the production of energy from fat, you distribute moderate amounts of energy over longer periods. Swimming, long-distance running and dancing are all aerobic activities. Sprinting, however, uses short bursts.

Aerobic exercises have many benefits. This is why doctors recommend them to patients regardless of their weight. These benefits include strengthening the repertory muscle, increasing oxygen and blood flow, and improving endurance.

There is no reason to avoid aerobics. There are many great programs that include both individual and group activities. Before you begin any type of new health care regimen, it is essential to understand how aerobics works. This can be done in many ways.

Talking to your doctor is the first step to making informed health decisions. Your doctor will tell you about programs that aren't beneficial to your body, too hard or could inflict injury. Your doctor will explain the best exercises and recommend personal trainers. They will also stress the many health benefits of aerobics. Your doctor should be your first stop. You should allow yourself enough time to ask any questions.

Information on aerobics can also be found online. The Internet offers many resources, including articles on its history and benefits. You can also interact with other users in chat rooms and forums to exchange experiences and answer questions. You can find information about specific routines on the Internet, and many websites will help you to put together routines that suit your level of experience.

You can also learn more about aerobics by reading the literature. You should find a wide range of books at your local library.

You can always go to the nearest bookshop if the materials are not up-to-date. Before you buy a book, make sure to check the internet for discounts.

These magazines can also be very valuable. Although the information may not be available to professionals, health care professionals have reviewed the articles in these magazines.

It is easy to learn about aerobics. It is easy to learn about aerobics.

Aerobics can reduce the risk of death from cardiovascular problems and prevent osteoporosis in men and women.

Regular exercise will help you to cope with the many challenges life brings. It will also help you to fight heart disease, lower your risk of developing osteoporosis, prevent breast and colon cancers, and reduce anxiety, stress, and anxiety. Aerobics is the key to a more productive and healthy life. Don't wait any longer to get started.

Exercise Is For Any Age Group

Everybody wants to be healthier. While this is true for all, there are some people who need to be careful about how they exercise to avoid injury.

These people include seniors. You should consider many things when it comes to aerobics. You must continue to build aerobic exercise. Depending on your health, you may need to start small. You need to start small, with the basics of work, in order to improve your health. Then, gradually move up to higher levels. This is particularly important for seniors. Before you start exercising every day, take a look at your health. Senior citizens are more likely to have health problems so it is important that they see a doctor immediately.

After getting cleared by a doctor, seniors are able to begin aerobic exercise as they would any other age. You can start by focusing on your goals in aerobics. An aerobic workout is beneficial as long as it's not too strenuous.

Remember to discuss your plans with your doctor, even if it is not a concern for you. Your doctor can give you more information on the type of exercise that is best for your needs.

Endurance and Intensity

Aerobics can help you lose weight and stay healthy. They strengthen your heart and breathing, and burn fat. Many people don't know how to exercise aerobically. For any exercise to be effective, intensity is key. Follow these guidelines to make sure you get the best results.

Find the level of intensity that you are comfortable with. You may get injured if you exercise too hard. You will not lose weight or get stronger if you don't work out enough. You need to find the right intensity program for you. Try to include enough weight or speed in any new exercise that you are trying. However, it shouldn't be too difficult. As your endurance and tolerance increase, you'll need to adjust the intensity of your workout. To make sure your workouts are still effective, check in on it every other week.

Safety is the second rule of intensity. Overtraining can be dangerous for you and your family. You may find that you are not getting the desired results and you might be tempted to increase your training. This is a good thing. However, if you do it too often, you could end up vomiting and possibly injuring yourself. Your muscles should feel sore if you're properly training, but your joints shouldn't.

Do not do a hard workout that makes it difficult to control your breathing or form. Take breaks, and then use slower speeds or lower weights to get back on track. This will allow you to get more from your workout. If you are injured during a workout, get help from those around you. It's always a good idea for you to partner up or take part in a class.

Finally, focus on intensity rather than jumping into the deep end. You won't be able run the London Marathon if you start exercising when you first begin. You can avoid injury and frustration by building up slowly. You will have more success if you slowly build up your exercise program.

It doesn't matter how good your current fitness level is, it's important to get better. People who haven't exercised in years or aren't in great shape often create aerobic workouts. There are also people who have done endurance work and want to create workouts. They are familiar with the basics of aerobics, and they simply want to help you get in shape.

Aerobic workouts are important if you've been exercising for a while or play a sport that requires endurance. Aerobics is a great way to increase your heart rate and breathe rate to get in shape. If you're an athlete, the basics class will be boring and not beneficial to you. There are many things you can do to get in shape.

The point of aerobics is to increase your heart rate and improve your breathing. If you're already an endurance athlete, this means you will need to find ways that you can push yourself beyond what you're capable of. You don't need to be a seasoned runner to run long distances.

To challenge your body, you need to make sure you have a variety of workouts. To challenge your body, you will need to speed up or add something.

Aerobic workouts are about challenging your body. You must find ways to make your body work harder.

Chapter 3: How to Create Your Amazing Home Gym

You will need to start by creating your own home gym. You will need to find the right equipment and stock up your home. This is what you should do.

Your workout goals and the end goal of your exercise program will determine what equipment you need. For example, the equipment that you use to lose weight and burn calories is different than what you would need to build muscle mass.

Building muscle is still one of the best ways to lose fat, as we'll see later in this book. Your metabolism will increase the more muscle you have.

You'll discover that there are certain principles and things that can be applied regardless of your goals. There are certain pieces of equipment that every person should have. Let's look at some of these items and how to approach it.

What makes a good home gym?

When you start building your home gym, you will face some new challenges. First, your home gym should not be too expensive. It can be tempting to buy everything you need, even if you aren't a pro at the gym.

You also need to consider how you will store your equipment. This is easier if you have a dedicated space for your gym. If you don't have a room dedicated to your gym, you should think about how to make it easy to disassemble and reassemble on cue. Or, perhaps, a small enough space that it doesn't matter that much.

You also need to be careful not to break any cabinets or damage any tables.

Start small, then work your way up. This means that you should only buy the essential items, but approach them in a way that allows you to grow and expand on what you have.

For example, take dumbbells. You can use dumbbells for almost any workout and they can reach all body parts. If you want to make a difference in your muscle growth, you will need dumbbells that can hold enough weight. The definition of "heavy enough" depends on how you move and your progress. Even for athletes who are trained, lateral dumbbell raises can be difficult with anything over 10 kg. However, dumbbell presses would require 10kg.

This is why it's a good idea to get dumbbells that are adjustable in size. You should be able remove or add weights as your situation dictates and build up. You can buy dumbbell sets starting at $30, which will allow you to increase your weight by up to 20kg. This is a good starting point. You might also want to purchase two dumbbell sets, which will allow you to increase your weight further.

This is only one example of how to approach your home gym modularly and compactly, saving money while still maximizing functionality. The pull up bar is another example. It is a very discreet item that costs only $10 and will not be noticed. Pull up bars are available that do not require drilling in the ground. They simply fit over your door frame to be fixed into place.

What is the best equipment to improve your pull-up bar? Gymnastic rings! Simply put, gymnastic rings are plastic rings that attach to rope. They can be looped over pull-up bars. These rings allow you to do ring dips and muscle ups. They are very affordable and can be stored in many places.

Skipping rope is an alternative to the treadmill. You can also use a bull worker, which is a piece made of metal that resists being squeezed. You can also do many things with everyday household items, as we'll see in the book.

You can think outside the box and use these tips to build a gym that does all you need without taking up too much space in your home.

These are the basics you should invest in

For those who want to know more, here are some equipment options that you can purchase over time. You will notice that these items are not essential for starting your gym, except for the pull-up bar and the dumbbells, depending on your goals and interests.

Here's how you can get started.

Pull up bar: A pull up bar, as mentioned above, is all you need to begin building and training muscle. This is because most muscles can be trained with bodyweight alone. You can train your chest, shoulders and abs by doing press-ups. Sit ups can also be used to train your abs.

The biceps, and the lats are the most difficult parts to train without equipment. These muscles are called 'pulling' and you must pull something to use them. You can't pull the floor towards you so you need to curl or hang.

A pull-up bar is a great tool for training your whole body. However, it's easier to get two or more items.

Dumbbells: Dumbbells can be used for so many purposes, beyond just bicep curls. You can use them for many other purposes, such as tricep presses and rows that work your lats. They can be used to increase your body's weight while you train your legs.

You should ensure that dumbbells can be lifted in weight. If you have good strength, you can start with 20kg and then buy two sets to increase your weight.

Bench: A bench is a great investment to help you take your training to the next step. You will be able to use dumbbells more efficiently, such as flyes, dumbbell presses, and other moves. An adjustable back bench is the best. This will allow you to sit or lie down on it, which will enable you to do isolation curls and other moves.

A bench that folds up can be a great option. You can store your bench underneath a bed or behind your wardrobe so it doesn't get in the way.

You will need an exercise mat. Although it isn't essential, you will notice that your floors can become slippery from sweating and cause a mess. A mat makes it much easier to do moves such as sit-ups, without putting pressure on your back or buttocks. It's also great for stretching, and other purposes.

Skipping rope: There are few better ways to burn calories than simply skipping rope.

Kettlebell: You're getting more advanced with your kettlebell. Kettlebells are great for training legs and burning calories. They will let you perform kettlebell swings as well as all kinds of squats, such goblet squats. You can increase your leg strength by using a bar for deadlifts or squats. This is good news because deadlifts and other squats require a lot space and can be difficult to set up. You can also use a kettlebell for functional strength exercises such as one-armed presses.

Gymnastic rings: We have already mentioned the incredible benefits of gymnastic ring. These will allow you to do the same exercises as TRX but at a fraction of the cost. They actually allow you to do more, as TRX isn't suitable for dips.

Bench Press: If you are serious about lifting weights, a bench press is a great investment. You will need to purchase a bar, which you may want to make permanent so you don't have to load and unload the bar each time you lift.

Chapter 4: Beginning

For total body fitness and health, full-body exercises are vital. Regular exercise is not only good for your health and well-being, but it will also improve your self-esteem, your relationships with others, and many other areas of your life. It is natural to get excited about starting a new exercise program, but you will also encounter some challenges. You will be surprised at how little you know about the anatomy of your body, how it develops after exercising, and the best way to exercise without equipment.

These stats show that regular exercise has many health benefits that will prove to be invaluable for those who are active in physical activity.

Reduced chance of getting a mental illness.

Colorectal Cancer: 50% less likely

Chances of suffering from stroke, heart disease or physical disability are decreased by 25%

- Premature death rates are reduced to 25%

You should also exercise for other reasons, not just those listed above.

- Regulation of blood sugar levels, insulin. The hormone insulin is made in the pancreas. Regular exercise helps to maintain a healthy sugar level and determine how effective insulin will be at controlling spikes or well-regulated sugar levels. Regular exercise can help to prevent type 2 diabetes and other metabolic diseases.

- Happy hormones are released when you exercise. This makes you feel good and calms you down. Do not set unrealistic goals for yourself. This can lead to depression and a feeling of inadequacy. Once you achieve your goals, your self-worth and confidence will increase. You will also be able handle more challenging workouts as you improve your endurance.

- Mental Alertness, Strength. When the body is exercising, the hippocampus (a part of the brain responsible for memory retention and information retention) becomes active. You need to be active to improve the function of your brain, and ultimately, your overall wellbeing.

- Reduces the risk of heart disease. When the body is engaged in controlled movements such as workouts, it is strengthened. This is because there is increased blood flow to the muscles which results in more oxygen being pushed to all parts of the body. Regular exercise reduces the risk of cardiovascular problems such as stress and other issues.

- Combating addiction. Workouts can help you get rid of the unhealthy attachment to drugs and other behaviors you struggle with. You will find that your mental energy is directed to positive endeavors and a decrease in addictions. Most likely, you won't experience withdrawal symptoms from cravings.

- Strengthening and developing the muscle. The right and well-planned form of exercises, which is appropriate for your body type and age, will increase muscle tone, strength, as well as general development. After the session, the body will start to replace and repair any muscle mass that is no longer functioning optimally. Muscle hypertrophy is the process that replaces the weakened muscle mass with new protein fibers. This can only be done if you are willing to put all your muscle mass to work.

Those who exercised before the lockdown were in effect can easily testify to how much it has improved their lives. They have found ways to overcome the sedentary lifestyle they lead these past weeks. You have missed a lot if you haven't started to exercise and your previous way of getting your body moving was by working around. However, you can and should start exercising in the comfort of your own home. You should aim to be able to do the exercises at a level that is comfortable for you and your body without putting too much stress on it. These workouts will build blocks that will help you to approach other areas of your life in positive ways.

Exercise: Brain and body response

You will notice a shift in your mental and physical health when you make exercise a regular part of your daily life. Strong evidence points to the positive effects of regular exercise. It is important to understand the interdependence between your mind, body and regular exercise. This will help you quickly understand and gain a full understanding of your body's response to exercise and stress. You will be able to identify the best workouts for yourself if you're an athlete with a lot of experience or someone who regularly exercises. For beginners, it is still possible to combine the best workouts for you, as long as you understand the connection between your mind and body.

Regular and coordinated movements of the muscular and respiratory systems of the body are required for a workout session. The duration and intensity of these sessions will depend on the individual's fitness. Your body will adapt to the repetitive motions of exercise if it is put through constant movements. Your body may find it difficult to perform the most basic movements at first because it isn't used to these activity levels. You will find that your body's ability to perform the basic movements is much better than it was a few weeks back if you do regular workouts without stressing your body. The speed at which the changes are apparent or how quickly your body adapts to them depends on how fit and how intense the exercise is. Your body will be able to handle the stress if you stick to your exercise schedule. The problem is that if you stop exercising, your body will no longer have the stimulation it needs. This can lead to a decrease in efficiency and a loss of ability for the body's ability to cope with stress levels that it might not have been able to handle before. Detraining is the phase in which your body stops exercising.

Your body adapts to exercise in stages. The first stage is known as the alarm or signal stage. This is your body's initial response when you start exercising. This is the initial response of your body to exercise. This is the resistance stage, where your body attempts to adapt to the environment. This stage is when the body's energy reserves are depleted and it is common for people to feel tired and fatigued. You can take palliative steps to reduce the intensity of this stage. These include breaking up your workouts into sets, resting, and making sure your diet is balanced with the right food classes. This will ensure that your body has the energy it needs and won't give up easily. This will allow you to exercise for longer periods without feeling fatigued.

It is important to include the brain in your workouts. The brain secretes essential growth hormones which promote muscle building. The brain is affected by the stress you experience while exercising. To help the body control stress levels, it produces stress hormones called Endorphins, Brain - Derived Neurotropic Factor (BNDF). This also helps to secrete other hormones that are essential for your physical and nervous health.

Chapter 5: Supermans

Step 1

Start Position: Lay on your stomach on a floor or mat with your legs extended behind you. Your toes should point toward the wall behind. Your palms are facing each other, so reach your arms up high.

Align your head and neck with your spine.

Step 2

Inhale. To stabilize your spine, strengthen your abdominal and core muscles. Slowly and steadily lift your legs off the ground until your legs are a few inches away from your torso. Keep both your arms straight and float them a few inches above the floor. You should keep your legs straight. Your head should be aligned with the spine. Your head should not lift off the ground or droop towards it. Don't allow your back to arch. This position should be held for a few seconds.

Step 3

Downward Phase: Inhale slowly and gently lower your arms and legs back to the starting position.

Push-Up

Step 1

Start Position: Place your hands on the mat in a hands-and-knees (quadruped) position. Your fingers should be facing forward. Engage your abdominals and draw the shoulder blades towards your back.

Step 2

You will reach one leg out, then the other. This will bring you to a plank position. Brace your torso by keeping the core/abs engaged. Your head should align with your spine. With your feet together, your toes should be tucked under your spine and your heels pointed toward the wall behind.

Step 3

Downward Phase: Slowly bend your elbows and lower your body towards the floor. Your torso should remain straight and your head should be aligned with the spine. Your hips should not be able to rise or fall, or your low back and ribcage should not sag. To maintain stability and a straight body, engage your glute (glutes), and quadriceps (quadriceps). Your chest and chin should touch the floor or mat. Your elbows should be kept close to your body, or you can allow them to flare slightly.

Step 4

Upward Phase: Straighten your elbows and press upward through your arms. Your torso should remain straight and your head should be aligned with the spine. Think of pushing the floor away. Don't allow your back to slump or your hips and hips to rise.

Step 5

Alternately, you can keep your fingers in front and your elbows near your sides during the down phase. This will shift the focus from the chest muscles to the triceps, which may decrease stress in the shoulder joint.

Pressing down on the heel and outside of your palm will increase your force and stability for your shoulders.

Contralateral Limb Raises

Step 1

Start Position: Lay on your stomach on a floor or mat with your legs extended behind you. Your toes should point toward the wall behind. Your arms should be extended overhead, your palms facing one another. Your head should be aligned with the spine.

Step 2

Inhale. To stabilize your spine, strengthen your abdominal/core muscles and slowly lift one arm off the ground. Your arm should be straight. Avoid rotating your shoulder or arm. Avoid any movement of your head or torso, and avoid arching in the back. Don't lift or lower your head. This position should be held for a few seconds.

Step 3

Downward Phase: Inhale slowly and gently lower your arm towards the starting position.

Step 4

Exercise Variation (1): Starting in a neutral position, strengthen your core and abdominal muscles to stabilize your spine. Next, slowly stretch your leg out and let it lift off the ground. Your leg should be straight, with your toes touching the wall behind. Keep your hip bones and pubic bone in direct contact with the mat. Avoid rotation of your pelvis or leg. Avoid any movement of your head or torso, and avoid arching in the back. Don't lift or lower your head. This position should be held for a few seconds. Restore your position.

Step 5

Exercise Variation (2): Starting in a neutral position, strengthen your core/abdominal muscles to stabilize your spine. Lift one leg off the ground by reaching out. The opposite arm should be positioned a few inches above the floor. You should keep your arm straight, and neither your leg nor your arm should rotate. Avoid any movement in your head or torso, and avoid arching your back. Don't lift or lower your head. This position should be held for a few seconds. Restore your position.

Pushups for the Bent Knee

Step 1

Start Position: Place your hands under your shoulders and place your knees on the mat. Engage your abdominals and draw the shoulder blades towards your back.

Step 2

As needed, reposition your knees to make a straight line through your body. This should be done from your knees through your torso through your head. The hips should not be bent. Keep your abdominals straight.

Step 3

Downward Phase: Keep your torso straight and your head aligned with the spine. Slowly bend your elbows to lower your body towards the floor. Your hips should not be raised or your lower back should not sag. Keep lowering your body until your chest and chin touch the floor or mat. Your elbows should not be too far from your body.

Step 4

Upward Phase: Keep your torso straight and your head aligned with the spine. Press upwards through your arms. Your hips should not be lifted upwards or your back should remain straight. Keep pressing until your elbows are straight.

Push-ups put stress on the wrist joints. You can reduce some of the stress by using dumbbells. Instead of putting your hands on the ground, grip the handles and use dumbbells. Pressing from an elevated position such as a dumbbell does not require you to lower your chest, or chin to touch the ground. Instead, lower yourself so that your chest and chin meet the dumbbell handles.

Dog that is downward facing

Step 1

Start Position: Place your hands on the ground and place your arms under your shoulders. To support your spine, engage your abdominals and step back one at a time. You will then reach push-up (plank) position. Your hands should be under your shoulders. To allow your feet to fully extend, reposition your feet. You should not allow your ribcage, low back or hips to sag towards the floor.

Step 2

Inhale. Your weight should be shifted back towards the wall behind. Your hips will rise in the air, creating an inverted V shape. Your head should be in line with your spine, or slightly tucked. Do not lift your head. Your heels should be pointed towards the floor. You may be able to bend your knees slightly if you have tight hamstrings. Keep your knees straight and point your heels towards the floor.

Step 3

Downward Phase: Take a deep breath and inhale. You should return to your starting push-up position.

Crunches

Step 1

Start Position: Lay on your back on a surface with your knees bent and your feet flat on the ground. Keep your heels about 12-18 inches from your seat.

Step 2

Your hands should be behind your head. Your elbows should be positioned behind your head. Throughout the exercise, you should keep your elbows straight. Your head should align with your spine.

Step 3

Inhale and move up to the upward phase. Engage your core and abdominal muscles. As you gently lift your head off the mat, chin a little. Your rib cage should be pulled together towards your pelvis. Relax your neck. At all times, your feet, tailbone, and lower back should be in direct contact with the mat. Keep curling until your upper back lifts off the mat. This position should be held for a moment.

Step 4

Downward Phase: Slowly and controlled, inhale slowly and lower your body toward the mat. Your feet, tailbone, and lower back should be in direct contact with the mat.

To avoid excessive strain on the low back, proper form is essential for this exercise. This movement is often performed too quickly and people may need to use the hip flexors for support in the upward phase. This can cause the pelvis tilt anteriorly and increase the strain on the low back. The abdominals are the link between the pelvis and the rib cage. Therefore, the movement should be focused on bringing the two parts together while keeping the neck relaxed.

Chapter 6: Questions to Ask Before You Start a Fitness Program

You are going to get fit and start exercising? Kudos to you! It is one of your best choices. Exercise is a great way to lose weight and keep fit. It also helps with heart disease, arthritis, depression relief, and other health benefits.

What do you do? Are you going to the gym? Do you want to try out different equipment? Are you going to start running in the morning? Will you use the treadmill that's been in your basement for years, or will you run?

These questions should be asked before you do these things or start a fitness program.

What are my fitness goals

Are you looking to lose weight? Are you looking to tone your body? Do you want to tone your muscles? It is important to know your goals and be clear about them. You need a plan and an end goal to be successful in any endeavor. You can then execute your plan and achieve success.

This will help you to see clearly what you want from your exercise program. This will help you choose the right type of exercise and equipment to use in order to achieve your fitness goals.

Are I able to do this?

After you have established your goals, it is a good idea to consult your doctor before you start your exercise program. This will ensure that you are fit enough to use the equipment you choose. Although exercise is generally good for your health there are some risks associated with physical stress. This applies to men and women aged 45 and 55, as well as those with certain medical conditions. Before you start an exercise program, get medical clearance from your doctor. While you're at it, ask your doctor for their advice on the best exercise equipment.

What time do I have?

You can achieve your fitness goals by dedicating your time to the exercises you love. To gain momentum in your fitness program, you must be consistent with how much time you spend on it. These are some questions to ask yourself: "How much time can I dedicate to exercise?", "Will my schedule accommodate this exercise program?", and "Am i willing to change my schedule to accommodate my exercise schedule?"

How can I stay motivated?

Exercise can be boring. Even if you exercise at home, it can be frustrating. It will be difficult to get up from the couch and move on to the treadmill at times. It will feel more productive to spend your time watching TV than finishing that Zumba DVD you just purchased. You can think of many excuses to not exercise. What can you do to stay motivated?

You need to think about the things that will motivate you long-term when you start an exercise program. Do you feel motivated to run if you can lose weight and become four sizes smaller? Do you feel lighter and more powerful? Does this motivate you to ride longer distances on your bike? Consider the motivations that you will use to keep exercising. These things can be written on a piece paper and posted on a wall or somewhere that is easily visible. This will help you to remember why you exercise each day.

You can also try something new. If you get bored, try different things. You can't do anything without consistency, even when you work out. Even if you only manage a small amount each day, make it count.

Chapter 7: The Three Most Important Rules For Body Transformation

Rule 1. Rule I.

You set goals and create a plan. You can move forward faster or slower by taking small steps. You will feel fulfilled and satisfied by your actions.

Setting goals is key to success. You lack direction and focus if you don't have goals. Setting goals allows you to be in control of your destiny and provides a baseline for measuring whether you're succeeding. Think about why you want something to change and what you will gain from it before you set yourself a goal. A sense of purpose can help you overcome obstacles. To achieve ambitious goals, we must work hard and be committed. We can therefore expect to face difficulties with its implementation sooner than later.

Setting goals is a process that allows you to define exactly what you want and when. This will help you to know which areas you should be focusing on and which ones you can let go. Be aware that a goal must have multiple key elements.

Write something now. Next, set your goal for the next pages. Be sure the goal is reachable. Your body can burn body fat and build muscle mass at about 2 pounds per week. Let goal setting be a challenge. For the next 8-10 weeks, set a goal. You can make a significant improvement in your appearance and develop positive habits during this period. You will experience an increase in energy and confidence. You will also notice that others notice your changes after 12 weeks. This will give you immense satisfaction and motivate you to take further action. You will achieve all of this if your persistence is strong. It is a good idea to ask yourself the following question: What are my goals for this year? After you have identified your goal, ask yourself the following question: What are my steps to reach it? Fill out the "Plan for action". I suggest that the plan be based on at least three aspects that will produce the best and most rapid results.

Your action plan for body transformation can be sequential. Regular training three times per week. Pre-determined caloric requirements, such as: Keeping to a strict diet for 8 weeks.

Next, set a date and a start date for each stage of your body transformation. Don't forget about rewarding yourself for any successes. Reward yourself for sticking to your plan for at least a week.

Another thing: be open to making mistakes. Even if your goal is lofty. It doesn't matter if your plan is perfect. There will be times when you have to make mistakes. You might leave training or eat too many sweets. You should not abandon your goal and not give up on it. We are all human, and we make mistakes.

Only one rule applies: Learn from your mistakes. What went wrong? What if you fail? Have you broken your pre-set rules? It happened. Find out the reasons why things didn't go your way. Keep going. Every step you take after a temporary failure will bring you closer to your goal. All of the above can be applied to any other area of your life.

Rule II. Rule II.

Calories simply represent energy. It is well-known that calories are a measure of energy.

You can track your calories and control your weight. You need to consume approximately 3,500 calories to lose 1 pound (0.45 kg) of body weight. It can take some time to count calories at the beginning. It will become easier as you go along. It's not something I do now. Let me tell you, it is worth starting at the beginning. Calorie counting is a great way to reduce overeating. It will give you an accurate picture of your actual calorie intake. For at least 21 days, count calories. You will soon become an expert and have control of your weight. This will mean that the trainer's assistance is no longer necessary.

If you consume more than 1000 calories per day than your daily caloric intake, you will gain 7000 calories each week. This gives us one kilogram (about 700gr pure muscle, the rest being glycogen and water).

This rate will allow you to gain approximately 7/8 pounds (4/5 kg) per month. This is a safe and healthy result. The first few weeks can see a rapid increase in kilograms due to an increase in water and muscle glycogen. To lose 1 kilogram (2 lb) of weight, you will need to eat less than 7000kcal. You can lose 500 kcal per day if you eat 500 kcal more each day and train intensely four times a week, burning 500 calories every training session. It gives us 5,500 calories per day, if we add it all. This pace will allow you to lose more than 3kg (6/7lbs) of body weight in one month. It is important to remember that even though you eat fewer calories, the body will still try to protect itself and slow down your metabolism. It is worth having a "cheat meal" at least once a week. This is a way to speed up your metabolism. You can afford higher calorie meals such as pizza, ice cream, or any other type of food. In a meal, it is crucial that complex and simple carbohydrates are balanced.

How to begin.

You will need to determine how many calories your body needs daily and how many calories you should consume to lose or gain weight.

What is BMR?

BMR is the Basal Metabolic Ratio. It calculates how many calories you would burn if you were not active and stayed in bed for the entire day. BMR calculator can be used to calculate the amount of calories you burn during inactivity and the daily calories. This takes into consideration your level of activity. These numbers give you a good idea of your daily calorie requirements.

Remember that basic metabolism calculations do not include lean body mass. This factor is also important. A calculation for basic metabolism will not take into account lean body mass. Overweight people will likely get a calculation that is too high.

How to calculate your BMR

Remember that basic metabolism (BMR) calculations for men and women are different. This is because men have more non-fat body mass (BMR) than women. There are easy methods and formulas that you can use to quickly calculate your BMR and daily calories. Take a moment to calculate your daily caloric requirements according to the following pattern.

These formulae can be used to calculate your BMR.

Men's BMR

BMR (metric formula) = (10 x weight per kg + (6.25x height per cm) + (5 x age over 5 years) +

BMR (imperial formula = 66.47) + (6.24x weight in pounds) + (12.7x height in inches) - (6.755x age in years)

BMR for women

BMR (metric formula) = (10 x weight per kg + (6.25x height per cm) - (5.25x age in years). - 161

BMR (imperial formula = 655.1 + (4.35x weight in pounds) + (4.7x height in inches) -(4.7x age in years)

Daily Calories Demand

Once you have developed BMR, you will be able to calculate your daily calories by adding BMR to one of these activity level factors:

Calories per Day = BMR x 1.

Active (light exercise, sports, 1-3 days per week) Calories per Day = BMR x 1.375

Moderately active (bicycling 3-5 days per week). Calories per Day = BMR x 1.55

You are active (heavy exercise for 6-7 days per week), Calories per Day = BMR x 1.75

You are more active (hard exercise or physical work), Calories per Day = BMR x 1.

Calorie Needs Daily

Now that you know how many calories are needed daily to maintain your weight, subtract 15-20% from the result. This will determine your surplus or deficit. It depends on what purpose you have. If you are obese, subtract calories from your daily requirements. If you are just thin and wish to gain weight, you can increase your calories. You should not exceed your BMR without taking into consideration the activity level.

To achieve your goal, you must eat a day.

kcal

This simple formula can be used to quickly lose weight if you are extremely obese. Important! Important!

Rule 3. Keep track of your progress

It is extremely helpful to track the effects. This will increase your chances of success by a large extent. Without a plan, it's not worth training. It's like having a map. You can track the results in your training journal and stick to your workout plan. Imagine that you have a goal for a city, but don't know how to get there. Navigation will guide you to your destination. The only thing you need to do is stay on the road and observe the signs. The same goes for your goal. You need to know what you want and how much weight you need to lose. You only need to follow a plan and keep track of your progress. You will reach your destination thanks to these steps. The only thing that remains is the time it will take to get there.

Research has shown that tracking your progress is a great way to track your progress and help you reach your goals. These are just a few of the reasons.

It Reminds you of Progress - Once you have established your baseline, you can keep track to measure the progress. It is important to celebrate your successes, no matter how small, in order to keep your motivation and confidence high. You can have something to celebrate, and it will push you to reach your goal.

Identifies Problems: People who track their progress know instantly when they have stopped making progress. It allows you to make course corrections. This allows you to determine what went wrong and why.

Focus Your Attention - People who track are able to stay on track due to the fact that they pay attention and focus their attention.

You can track your progress and stay focused on the important things that will help you reach your goals. It can help you identify obstacles and develop strategies to overcome them. It helps you to set realistic goals and keep your eyes on the prize.

No matter how many times you log your data, the workout log provides positive reinforcement. You will also get a boost by tracking your progress over time. You know that you have achieved something when you are able to do 70 push-ups compared to 30 push-ups two months ago.

A diary helps you stay motivated and also records your workouts. Your workout log may be a clue to why your weight training isn't working.

Chapter 8: Basic Stretching

Stretching and mobilizing the muscles and joints before you jump into a hard workout is a good idea.

This is a basic, but effective, full-body mobilization and stretching routine you can do before starting a workout. Take a minute to learn each stretch according to the instructions below.

Head tilts

For 3-4 seconds, tilt your head slowly from side to side, forward and back. Keep it in the full tilt position (stretching).

Arm swings

Standing, extend your arms straight out and keep them parallel to the ground. Start making small circles with your arms straight. Slowly increase your circle radius by swinging your arms in a windmill-style motion. Change the direction of your circles by going backwards. Slowly make the circles smaller, until your arms meet the ground. Continue to change direction until your shoulders feel warm.

Shoulder Stretch Behind-the Head

Place your right hand on your right shoulder and extend your elbow towards the ceiling. Next, extend your left elbow towards the left by gently extending your left elbow. Keep doing this until your elbow is fully extended. You can do the same for the other arm.

Double shoulder stretch

Keep your fingers together in front of yourself. Next, extend your palms to the ceiling with full extension. Focus on stretching your shoulders as high as you can. For 4 to 5 seconds, hold.

Cross the chest shoulder stretch

Your left arm should be crossed in front of you towards your right side. Slowly squeeze your left elbow towards your right shoulder by grabbing your right elbow with your right hand. This should be done for approximately 5 seconds. You can do the same for the opposite side.

Behind the Shoulder Stretch

Your left arm should be behind your back, with your forearm horizontal to the ground. Take your left hand and pull it towards your right. As you pull your left hand over, gently lift it by moving it slightly upwards. This will increase the stretch in your shoulder. You can hold the position for 7 to 8 seconds. Then, see if you are able to go an inch further! You can do the same for the opposite side.

Back Rotations

Standing with your feet shoulder width apart, your arms outstretched sideways parallel to the ground, your legs straighten slightly. To increase momentum, rotate your hips as far as possible to the left. Use your arms to move your arms. To increase momentum, spin your body through the center point to the opposite extreme. Once you are at full rotation, use your arms to help propel the spin. Repeat this process until your back feels loose.

Hamstring Stretch

Place your feet together and stand straight. Keep your legs straight and your arms straight. Now, extend your hands towards the ground. As you reach the end of the stretch, exhale. Touch the floor using your tips of your fingers. If that is possible, you can then flatten your hands on the ground. You should hold the stretch for 7 to 8 seconds.

Quad Stretch

To stabilize your balance, stand straight and grab a sturdy object such as a doorpost or wall to hold you upright. To catch your right foot, swing your right foot forward to reach your butt. Keep your knee under your body, and lift your foot as far as you can. Your quad muscles should be stretching. You should hold the stretch for seven to eight seconds. Continue with the other leg.

Hip Flexor Stretch

When you sit on an office chair, the hip flexor is the part that folds under the table. You should stretch this area before you do any exercise. There are many hip exercises that call for action from the hip joint. Standing straight, extend your legs as far as possible behind you. Keep your knees on the ground and your rear leg extended. Next, cross your fingers and reach your palms towards the ceiling. Keep your hips closer to the ground by extending your rear leg. Each leg should be held for approximately 10 seconds. You should keep your hips straight and not let your rear leg trail.

Groin Stretch

Place your feet on the ground and bring your feet together so your soles are against one another. Keep your feet as close to the ground as you can while holding your feet with your hands. Slowly squeeze your knees towards the ground by extending your elbows. When you have reached your maximum stretch, lean forward until your chest is fully extended. For about 10 seconds, hold the stretch. Now, take a deep breath and push your elbows down slightly. Next, lean forward with your chest. For another 3 to 5 seconds, hold this position. Relax and breathe in. Slowly get up.

Squat Stretch

Keep your feet shoulder width apart and lower your body into a squat position. Your butt should be as close as your heels. To keep your balance, you can lean forward onto your toes and feet to maintain balance. This is a stretch, not a strict squat. To help you keep your balance, you may need to place yourself near a wall or table. Keep your balance in the same area. Now, slowly move your butt towards your left foot and then towards your right foot. Continue this process several times until you feel comfortable in this position. You can add two more things to this position: (1) Move left and right while you are moving; (2) Next, place your elbows inside your knees and fold your hands in half. Use your elbows to push your knees forwards. Continue to stretch your muscles, tendons, and ligaments until you feel comfortable.

Inch Worms

Keep your feet together and lower your hands towards the floor. This is similar to the "Hamstring Stretch." Next, place your weight on your hands and "walk" your hands forward until your hands are in push-up plank position. Then, reverse the direction of your handwalk until your hands are directly in front of you feet. Repeat this process several times until your joints feel comfortable and warm.

Once you feel comfortable, move forward with your hands to push your hands up to the push-up plank position. Then, reverse the direction to your feet.

Foot Rotations

Keep one leg extended, and your foot off the ground. Rotate your foot as wide as possible for 7 rotations. Then reverse the direction of your rotation and repeat the process for the remaining 7 rotations. Do the same with the other foot.

Calf Stretch

Place your hands on a wall, and lean forward against the wall. To stabilize your weight, move your feet backwards and pick one foot. The other can be left free for now. Slowly, stretch your heel towards the floor while keeping your toes pointed at the wall. You should feel a stretch in your calf. You should keep the stretch going for 8-10 seconds. Next, change the angle of the toes so that your ankle and calf muscles are stretched slightly from different angles. Turn your side!

Chapter 9: Arms and Love Handles

We have covered two types of exercises you can do to get a lean, ripped body in the preceding chapters.

However, there are those who want to target particular areas of their bodies, such as their arms or lower back fat. This chapter will provide 5 of the best exercises for these areas.

Dips

Dips are one of the best exercises for getting your arms toned. You will notice a difference in your triceps and be able to achieve toned muscles quickly.

How to do: Dips can be performed on a chair or couch, but they should be sturdy. Place your palms facing the opposite direction on the couch or chair. Now, lift your butt off the chair. Your heels should support your body. Your lower torso should be moved by pushing your butt upwards and downwards. Your hands should move your upper torso. Continue to push your butt up and down until you feel the heat in your arms.

How many reps? You can do 20 or more reps, and up to 3 sets depending on your comfort level.

Pros: Many women find the triceps and arm area problematic. They are unable to lift heavy objects with their hands or use them for heavy-duty tasks. These areas will store extra fat, so it is important to target them. This will help you get positive results quickly by engaging all your muscles.

Pull ups

Pull ups can be used to strengthen your arms and lower back. This is your one-stop shop for all things arm strengthening.

How to do: You can perform regular pull-ups by placing a rod at a suitable level or using the edge of a table. To help your triceps, hold the rod in your hands. To make it easier for yourself, pull yourself up using force. However, you should cave in your body a bit, starting at your feet. Slip under the table and then pull yourself up.

To tone your biceps, you can hold the rod/table so that your fingers face you. There is very little space between your arms. Now, raise your head and touch the rod with both of your chins.

How many reps? Pull-ups can be difficult and it will take some time for your body adapt to them. Once you're able to pull up, you can do between 10-12 reps and 4 sets of each depending on how comfortable you are.

Pros: This exercise is great to strengthen the arms and upper body.

Pushups

Pushups can be as effective as pull-ups, and they will make your arms feel the burn.

Perform a push-up by standing with your legs together and your hands at your sides. To walk forward, squat down and use your hands. Your upper body should be supported by your hands, and your lower body should be supported with your toes. Now, bend your elbows so that your chest touches the ground. Next, bend your elbows so that you can touch the floor with your chest.

How many reps? This exercise is very easy. You can do 20 reps or 3 sets, depending on how comfortable you are.

Pros: Pushups are good for your core and arms. Pushups can be done every day to get slim arms.

Side planks

We looked at planks and learned about their benefits in chapter 1. This chapter will show you how side planks work and what they can do for your arms.

How to do: To perform a side-plank, first lie on your back and then move to your side. Use your right forearm to push your body upwards and balance your lower body with your feet. You can push your body upward and downward, and raise your left leg if necessary. To complete the side plank, you can do it again.

How many reps? You can do 20 or 3 sets, depending on how comfortable you are.

Side planks are a great way to work your thigh muscles, as well as your internal and external obliques. You will feel the heat in your active hand.

Arm circles

Arm circles are a great way to relax your arms and absorb the benefits of the rest. This is a great way to end your routine.

How to do it: Stand with your legs together and extend your arms outwards. These should be at the shoulder level. Start to rotate them clockwise. Keep the motion steady. Then, flip them clockwise. Keep going until your muscles tone up.

How many reps? You can do this for five minutes, and then take a break for a minute.

The pros: Although this exercise is easy, it will help to tone your arms.

Chapter 10: Doing Aerobic Exercise at Home: What Are the Wonders?

Are you looking to lose huge amounts of calories? Aerobics can be a great way to reach your fitness goals. You can even do it in your own home. Most people will dance the house while listening to their favorite music. This can be done in a variety of ways.

Aerobic exercise is also known as cardiovascular training. It involves a rhythmic activity that uses large muscle groups. Aerobic exercise has been proven to be a great way to lose weight, especially because it can be done at any hour of the day.

You can also walk, jog or climb stairs at home. This gives your body a much-needed workout. These can be done for as long as you are willing to work hard enough. You'll find your heart beat faster and your breathing speed increases.

How to train

Aerobic exercise should be done at least three times per week, for 30 to 60 minutes. You should start slowly. Do not try to go all out if you've been living a very sedentary life for a while. A 10-minute session will suffice if you feel that aerobics is too strenuous for you. Gradually increase your pace over the next few weeks until you feel comfortable exercising longer. You should slow down, but listen to your body. You can eliminate the chance of getting hurt.

Utilize Your Surroundings

Working out at home has the advantage of allowing you to use all available space for your workout.

Living room - This is where most people do their aerobic exercise. You can set the tone by playing the role. Play some music and dress up as if you're going to the gym. This will increase your motivation to exercise more and make you feel better. You will feel more motivated and get your adrenaline pumping.

Your own space - Exercise at home is a great way to keep your privacy, especially if it's in your own bedroom. You can avoid distractions like household chores or snooping relatives.

Garage - Invite friends over to use your garage for an hour of intense aerobics. To avoid any injuries or accidents, make sure that all cars are parked outside.

Warning! Before you start exercising, please read this warning.

Remember to warm up your muscles before you begin any exercise, even if you are not supervised by a trainer. Light calisthenics, easy stretching and a few minutes of cardio are some ways to prepare for exercise.

Aerobics with Low Impact

This type of aerobics is best for seniors, pregnant women, and overweight people. This type of aerobics is for people who want to get a routine that isn't too intense and who are looking to do a variety of movements before moving on to more intensive exercise.

How do you do it?

You can do a variety of movements. You don't have to follow a specific order. For starters, you can move forwards and backwards while simultaneously swinging your arms sideways. Each motion should be performed for at least a minute before you move on to the next.

Perform the same movements throughout your entire workout routine. These movements can be performed while you are warming up, cooling off, or in between more difficult motions.

What are some low-impact aerobic exercise options?

Heel Digs

This is one of the most popular aerobic exercises that you can do at your home. This is so easy that you only need to extend your legs forward. Tap each foot on the ground by extending your legs to the beat of the music. You can do the same thing with the other leg. Either swing your hands, or hold them in place. You can either swing your hands or keep them in place during this exercise. Your goal is to engage your muscles and not rely on gravity.

Duck Walks

It's more like walking in place, except that your legs are bent at your knees. Do the duck walk while pumping your arms in a controlled way. This aerobic exercise will help burn your thighs. Tip: To eliminate back pain, keep your back straight while you bend.

The Grapevine

The grapevine is another popular aerobic move. As you take a broad step to the right, bring your right foot towards the left and cross it behind your left foot. As you continue to move, bring your left foot up to stand. Then bring your right foot up to tap the left foot. Continue the process.

Grapevine is incomplete without arm movement. Slowly raise your arm up to the sides and then lift it above your head. Next, place your right foot behind you left. You can repeat the same process with your feet and arms.

Aerobics with High Impact

People who are healthy and in good physical condition should consider this. Health experts say that people who exercise regularly are more likely to have stronger bones and a healthier body. High-impact aerobics makes the heart pump harder, and helps shape muscles.

How do you do it?

You would perform low-impact aerobics in a similar way. However, your movements must be created and performed at a fast pace. Start your movements by moving in place. Warm up the same way as low-impact aerobics. This will prepare you for a more intense workout.

What are some high-impact aerobic exercises that you can do?

Jog in a Place

Your normal jogging can be made more challenging by elevating your knees as you jog. Alternate high-knee and normal jogging are also options. This will allow you to maintain your heart rate without getting exhausted.

Grasshopper Jump

This can be quite challenging for people with weak joints. You may need to exaggerate this type of jump. Standing, extend your left foot sideways and jump to the right. Return to your starting position and land with your feet crossed. You can repeat the same motion but now jump to your left.

Ski Jump

You will need to start in a similar position as skiing. You can start the routine by jumping up, with your knees bent and your torso slightly forward. Start by jumping up to your right side, ensuring that you land on both feet. Continue the same motion, jumping from the right to the left.

Chapter 11: The Benefits of Staying Fit

Knowing the benefits of an activity will give you the impetus to keep going. These are the benefits of a home workout program.

Protects Muscle Loss

As you age, it is no surprise that your body may not be as efficient as it once was. It becomes harder to build muscles and your muscles will start to break down quicker. It is no surprise that people who are older look less attractive. They look like beautiful flowers that lose their beauty. They eventually become stale.

Plan for regular exercise is a way to prepare for the later years of your life. However, planning is not enough. You must actually execute your plans. Regular exercise is essential for healthy aging. Regular exercise helps to increase and maintain muscle mass. People who looked strong and active into their later years might be something you have seen. It is possible to be as active and strong as that by exercising.

Regular exercise increases your metabolism and helps you to be more resilient in your daily activities. As you age, you will need the support of those around you. Working out can reduce your dependence on others. It also helps older adults avoid falling unconsciously.

Improves Digestion

Regular exercise can be beneficial for your overall health and digestion. If you make it a habit to exercise, your digestive system will be healthier and more robust. The gut is also healthy when you do physical activities. Your intestinal flow slows down if you are less active. Experts agree that exercising has both short-term as well long-term benefits.

It can also relieve gas, heartburn, constipation and stomach cramps. It is important to note that too many or poorly timed activities can cause digestive problems. You may experience stomach problems like constipation, heartburn and stomach pain. These issues can occur if you exercise immediately after eating. It is better to exercise before you eat than after.

It is possible to exercise after eating. It is all about the timing. It is important to exercise after eating. This is because blood flows around the stomach and intestines, which aids in digestion. If you do not allow your body to rest after exercising, blood can flow back to your stomach, muscles, and cause digestion problems.

Enhances Appearance

There are many ways that working out can improve your appearance. You can make your face look younger by strengthening your muscles and improving the quality of your skin. Regular exercise helps to rid your skin of oil and dirt. How do you detox your skin? How? You might not require a detoxifying drug if you exercise.

Audrey Kunin, a Kansas City dermatologist, said that regular exercise is like a mini-facial. According to her, sweating out can help eliminate the oil and sweat trapped in your pores. She recommends that you wash your face right away after you are done sweating. You can let the gunk build up in your pores if you don't do this.

Regular exercise is a great way to reduce stress and look younger. The aging process is accelerated by mental and physical exhaustion. You can give yourself a more youthful outlook if you start and maintain a workout program. You will also notice a difference in your appearance when you put on your workout clothes.

Increases mental performance and work productivity

To succeed in mentally demanding tasks, you need to be calm and relaxed. In today's digital world, this mental state is essential. To be your best, it is important to stay focused when working. You may be distracted because you're not relaxed. Regular exercise will give you the peace and tranquility that you need to succeed in daily activities.

Greater relaxation leads to greater efficiency. You cannot reach the top of your career and fulfill your potential if you are prone to poor performance. Because of the competitive nature of modern work, there's a lot of pressure on you to perform well or be fired. Many people are waiting to step in and take over your job. To be a successful entrepreneur, you must remain at the top of your game. You must be a competitive entrepreneur in order to survive the fierce business world. Exercise and other stress-relieving activities can give you the edge to be clear-headed.

Create a new circle of productive friends

To keep your sanity intact and reach your full potential, you need positive energy. In a world filled with negative influences, it is crucial to maintain the right company. There are many people who are interested in things that don't produce results, such as talking poorly about others or spending too much time on digital devices.

You can also choose to spend your time doing things that will improve your performance and health. You will attract the people you like. You'll find people you share the same interests as you and you will easily form friendships. You'll find it easier to make friends with people who enjoy working out and those who are more productive.

Joining a health club makes it easier to make friends with these people. This is because you are doing health-enhancing activities. You can find others who are doing the same thing by working out. They will help you improve your performance and can give you some tips to make you more efficient.

Alternatives to Social Media Activities

A positive habit can be a great way to stop a bad habit. You might be depressed because you are addicted to a substance that makes you happy. You might find that having hobbies or engaging in sports can make you happier than drug abuse.

You might also be addicted to digital devices, as that is what you do with your free time. You can get rid of it by engaging in productive activities like visiting loved ones and playing sports. A home workout program is another way to make time for your mental and physical health.

Chapter 12: Why you should be working out

Your diet and how you adjust to it will play a major role in your weight loss. Your body's shape will change only if you exercise. Your body will not shrink if you don't engage in cardiovascular activities or muscle building exercises. However, it will likely be smaller and less defined.

You're probably reading this book to shed weight and achieve the body you have been dreaming of. Regular exercise should be part of your daily routine, regardless if you are trying to lose 50 pounds or more or if you want to achieve a certain percentage (hoping to lose those annoying 10-15 pounds). Cardiovascular exercise, also known as cardio, is a great way to make your body healthier. Strength training, on the other hand, can help you look more attractive. Combining the two is a winning combination. Combine cardio and strength training with healthy eating habits, and your body will look and feel amazing.

Also, you will notice a change in your mood and energy. Exercise can influence how certain chemicals affect the brain. Being active on a regular basis can increase happiness in your daily life, without getting too technical. Although it is not a panacea, you may notice a decrease in stress levels. You may find that you aren't as depressed now as you used to be. You will feel more rested and have more energy for tomorrow. These positive changes will be noticed in your life and around you. You've made it a habit to be active every day.

However, it is not a relationship that will automatically blossom between you and your exercise. You're more likely to dislike exercise the first time you start. You might find it strange. You might feel uncomfortable. You might discover parts of your body - muscles or joints - you didn't know you had. Your brain will continue to search for better ways. Although you will have to fight and throw tantrums [with yourself, and with yourself], if you persevere through the difficult habit-building days, your brain will be able to see the pros.

Your quality of life will be improved by exercising. Regular activity is better if you begin to incorporate it into your daily life sooner than later. Although you may not see any changes right away, once you reach a certain point in your health journey, you will realize that it is a great decision. You feel great! That's the goal. You want to have a great body and look good. Those things won't compare to the emotions you'll feel when you look at the positive changes you've made inside and outside.

There is no reason to delay. Get started today!

This Home Workout

We've discussed diet. We have discussed the importance and benefits of exercising. Here are the benefits of this exercise that I created specifically for you. It may seem strange that he knows what you need, even though we have never met. This program is for me." The short answer to your question is yes. This program is 100% for you, and I'll tell you why.

This 28-day Lose Weight & Feel Great program will work regardless of where you live, what equipment is available, and what your fitness level. Whatever avenues you take to build muscle and work the heart, one thing is constant: the body. Cardiovascular health and weight lifting are not something that happens by itself. Physical presence is essential. This is the most important requirement for any exercise. Other things are optional. Shoes? They are optional, depending on what type of exercise you do. What about a shirt? Optional. Shorts? You can opt for shorts, but you will need them if you are in public. Do you have a weight bench or a treadmill? Optional

Let me explain. Your body was designed to be self-sufficient. Your body is your gym. It's also a free gym! Push ups. Sit ups. Squats. All of them require one thing: your body. Your body has its own weight. Your treadmill is where you are, wherever you go. You already have all the tools you need to achieve your highest physical condition, and I would love to help you.

It's possible you also guessed it! You don't need any equipment to reach your goals. Your body is the best exercise system. You can take it with you everywhere, you know the equipment well, and there is no waiting in line to use it.

We're ready to get started now that you are pumped up. You can find out more about my workout terminology in the next section. This section will help you to understand how to do your workouts.

Terminology for Workouts

Many fitness trainers will use abbreviations and acronyms. I'm no different. EXCEPT, I will tell you what they are so that you don't get lost during your workouts.

These are the terms that you will see most often in your exercise schedule.

AMRAP (as many repetitions possible) - Complete as many repetitions within a time limit.

Sets are a group that has multiple repetitions. For example, 3 sets of 10 burpees means 10 burpees followed by a brief rest. Then, 10 burpees and 10 more burpees. Complete the set with 10 burpees.

EMOM (Every minute on the Minute) - Perform exercises every minute for the time prescribed

Time is limited, so do as many repetitions/sets of each item as you can in the time allotted.

Ladder (set). An ascending/descending number of repetitions for multiple sets. (Example: 15 burpees and rest, 14 burpees and rest, 13 burpees and rest, 13 burpees, rest), 12 burpees, rest, 11 burpees, rest)

21-15-9 - Perform 21 repetitions for each exercise, then 15 repetitions for each exercise. Finally, perform 9 repetitions of each exercise. The entire cycle should be completed three times.

28-Day Workout Program

Here it is! Notice that the schedule does not start on a specific day of the week. There is a reason why. You don't have to wait until a specific day to start. You should begin immediately if you have decided that you are going to seriously take this challenge, regardless of whether it is Wednesday, Thursday, Monday, or

Tuesday. No delays! The first day of your 28 day schedule starts on the day that you choose. This is your workout.

The 28-day workout program is followed by several pages that include photos and descriptions for each exercise.

Exercise Guide

Suggestions for Supplements

Nutrition is key to weight loss. It is important to have the right nutrients for your diet. You also need top-quality nutrients to replenish your body after a workout. These dietary requirements could make the difference between your success and failure.

Optimum Nutrition is a popular brand in the supplement industry because of several reasons. Quality is the main reason. Optimum Nutrition offers the best quality protein at the most affordable price. It does not contain any fillers like other brands. Optimum Nutrition products are safe and effective, so you can rest assured that your body will get the best results.

My Personal Review

I have used Optimum Nutrition's whey proteins for over 5 years and have never had a negative experience. I have tried many different supplements in my career, but I always return to Optimum Nutrition.

Taste & Mixability (9/10).

You're familiar with the importance of taste and mixing ability in protein shakes. It's not fair to expect something delicious. Optimum Nutrition has a range of flavors, including vanilla, chocolate, strawberry banana, and many others. They taste just like milkshakes and I am surprised they are good for you. The powder can be mixed with 250ml water in a shaker. Give it a few shakes to dissolve completely. This supplement will not leave any powdery bits in your mouth.

Ingredient Profile (9/10)

You can't go wrong when you choose Optimum Nutrition whey proteins. They offer 24 grams of protein per serving. Optimum Nutrition whey proteins are 100% pure, real, and honest-to-goodness whey protein, unlike other supplement companies. The whey protein will be absorbed faster and more efficiently, which means it will result in faster recovery and protein synthesis. It also contains only 1 gram sugar. This makes it the perfect choice for people who are trying to lose weight. Protein shakes are often flavored with more sugar than necessary, which completely negates their purpose.

Optimum Nutrition whey proteins also contain essential amino acids (EEAs). Because the body can't create them naturally, these essential amino acids are vital. This is why the term, ESSENTIAL is necessary. EEAs can only be obtained through your diet. The best thing about including them in your protein shake is that they can increase muscle mass and, consequently, raise metabolism. What does this all mean? This means you will burn more calories every day, even when you are sleeping. Amazing!

Effectiveness (9/10).

You won't get a rush of energy from a protein shake. A protein shake's main purpose is to provide more protein and supplement your diet. It also helps to repair damaged muscles. Although I do not recommend supplements as a rule, I know of no one in the fitness world who doesn't drink protein shakes. Optimum Nutrition, as I mentioned earlier, is known for making quality supplements.

I have noticed an increase in strength, lean muscle mass, and recovery when I drink Optimum Nutrition whey proteins.

Value (9/10).

Optimum Nutrition offers a variety of whey protein options in different amounts. If you exercise every day, I believe you should consume at least one scoop per day. A 2 lb protein tub will last you about a month if you only plan to have one scoop per day.

Optimum Nutrition 2LB Whey Protein has 26 scoops (32g per rounded scoop), and is priced at Canadian $47.00+. This is $0.55+cents per scoop. This is a great deal compared to leading companies that usually cost $0.70+cents per scoop. This is how you should think about it. Is it healthier/cheaper/smarter to consume a protein shake with high quality nutrients that will keep your body fuller longer; costing only $0.55 a scoop, or would you prefer to purchase a BigMac combo at

McDonalds; selling for close to $6 or $7, fueling your body with low-quality nutrients that will leave you hungry again just after a couple of hours? Can you see the point?

Chapter 13: 30-Day Workout Challenge

We now come to the 30-day program. This program is an incremental one. You will start with lower intensity and do fewer reps. However, as your strength and stamina improve, you will be able to do more reps at a higher intensity.

You won't have to do it all at once. There will be days when you are able to take a break and you will have full rest days. Do not let your diet slip during these days. Keep up your daily stretching.

The program is primarily focused on strength and muscle toning exercises. However, the program also includes a few days for stamina/cardio exercises like running, walking and cycling. This will give you variety and ensure that you don't neglect any aspect of your fitness.

You will feel unable to go on if you don't exercise regularly. It is normal to feel discouraged at times. Keep your eyes on the prize - this is what you're doing for yourself. Your motivation must come from within. You will succeed if you believe in yourself

Day 1

10 sit-ups

10 push-ups

10 squats

Day 2

15 sit-ups

10 leg raises

10 squats

30-second plank

Day 3

15 push-ups

10 crunches

15 leg raises

Day 4

REST DAY

Day 5

15 sit-ups

15 crunches

15 squats

40-second plank

Day 6

20 push-ups

15 crunches

15 leg raises

50-second plank

Day 7

25 squats

15 sit-ups

20 leg raises

60-second plank

Day 8

REST DAY

Day 9

50-minute brisk walk

Day 10

5km jog OR

10km cycling

Day 11

30 push-ups

20 crunches

20 squats

70-second plank

Day 12

30 squats

20 crunches

25 leg raises

80-second plank

Day 13

30 sit-ups

25 crunches

25 leg raises

90-second plank

Day 14

REST DAY

Day 15

30 sit-ups

25 push-ups

30 leg raises

100-second plank

Day 16

30 sit-ups

30 crunches

30 leg raises

110-second plank

Day 17

35 squats

30 crunches

30 push-ups

120-second plank

Day 18

REST DAY

Day 19

35 sit-ups

35 crunches

35 leg raises

130-second plank

Day 20

40 sit-ups

35 push-ups

35 leg raises

140-second plank

Day 21

40 sit-ups

40 crunches

35 leg raises

150-second plank

Day 22

REST DAY

Day 23

22 jumping jacks

22 squats

22 push-ups

22 leg raises

Day 24

25 jumping jacks

25 sit-ups

25 push-ups

25 leg raises

Day 25

50-minute brisk walk

Day 26

5km jog OR

10km cycling

Day 27

45 squats

45 crunches

45 push-ups

160-second plank

Day 28

50 leg raises

50 crunches

45 push-ups

170-second plank

Day 29

30 jumping jacks

30 push-ups

30 squats

Day 30

50 sit-ups

50 push-ups

50 squats

180-second plank

Chapter 14: Bodyweight Exercises for Easy Weight Loss

Do you really need to lose weight? As you pass the gym, you think about joining. You might also consider purchasing a few pieces of exercise equipment and then using them at home. You don't need either one of these. You need Bodyweight. The best way to lose weight is by losing bodyweight. You only need to invest your time and not money.

It is much more difficult to lose weight than lifting weights or running on the treadmill at the gym. These exercises will improve your strength and help to tone your muscles, but they are not as effective as weight lifting or going to the gym. Traditional weight lifting only targets one muscle group at once. For example, bicep curls are a traditional exercise that targets your biceps. The chest is worked by bench pressing, but the lower body is not.

Although weight training is beneficial and has its advantages, bodyweight is far more effective in burning fat. It doesn't matter which Bodyweight exercise you choose, they all target multiple muscle groups simultaneously, making it one of the best methods to lose fat. Here are some common Bodyweight exercises that can help you lose fat.

Upper Body Exercises

Although these are intended to target the upper body, they will still need to use many other muscle groups in order to be effective.

Standard Push-ups

Although pushups are not something that anyone enjoys, they are essential for fat loss and strength. Push-ups are a very popular exercise in any fitness program. There is good reason why. Push-ups are not only good for your upper body (chest, shoulders and triceps), but also work your core muscles to prevent sagging.

Face down, lay flat on the ground.

Place your hands on the ground directly below your shoulders. Now, raise your arms up and place your hands flat on your stomach.

Your back should be straight, your feet must be together (easier), or you can set your feet apart (easier).

Bring your elbows to the floor by lowering your head until your chest touches it. Then, push yourself back up.

Begin with 5-10 reps, then increase your effort.

Decline Push-ups

These are more difficult than regular pushups because they require a wider range of movement. You can do the push-ups in the same way as a pushup, but elevate your feet by using a bench or chair. Your upper body should be lowered to the floor. Then, push up using your chest, shoulders, and triceps. Keep your spine straight, and your abs tight.

Spiderman Push-ups

This will make you feel like a super hero! This push-up is more difficult than any other type of push-up. You will feel like a superhero!

For a push-up, start in the standard position

Your chest should be lower than your elbows. At the same time, your right knee should be lifted towards your right elbow. Keep it simple and do it in one motion.

Lift your leg up and return it to its original position.

Next time, place your left knee on your left elbow.

Keep your stomach in a straight line, keep your back straight, and don't twist your hips.

Shoulder Press Push Up

This one is for you.

You will need to be in a position to do an elevated push-up with your feet on a bench. Now, move your hands closer to the bench and form an inverted V shape.

You have the option to bend or straighten your legs, depending on what is most comfortable.

Your head should be lowered to the ground. Then, push your chest up with your shoulders, chest and triceps.

Pull-Ups

As you use all your weight, these are one of the most important exercises to build strength.

Grab a bar that is fixed above your head with an overhand grip

Without straining, lift your body as high as possible without straining.

Slowly lower your back

Lower Body

There are many highly active muscles in your lower body that are constantly used throughout the day. Walking requires you to use your quadriceps muscles, calf muscles and hamstrings. Lower body exercises are essential to maintain your muscles' strength and health so that they can continue to support and work with you as well as shed some fat.

Squat

Because it works the lower part most, the squat should be a key component of any exercise program.

Place your feet slightly wider than shoulder width apart and stand with your feet slightly wider than your shoulders

Keep your abs tight and squeeze your glutes. Make sure your toes face forward.

Lower your body to the ground, but don't let your back go. Keep your knees straight.

Push your bottom back like you're tapping against a table. Never, ever arch your back or round your back. You will strain yourself.

For a return to normal, you can use your quadriceps, glutes, and hamstrings as a push-up.

Prisoner Squat

You can do a regular squat but instead of allowing your arms to hang by your sides, you should place your hands behind your head. You can eliminate some of the momentum you use in a regular squat by placing your hands behind your head. You are also adding weight to the equation by raising your hands. You should maintain the same form you do with a regular squat, but don't allow your hands to drop.

Y Squat

The Y squat looks similar to a prisoner's squat, but instead of holding your hands behind you, raise your arms up so that your arms are in a Y position over your head. Keep your shoulders straight and your back tense. When you squat, push your hips forward, backwards, and lower. Keep your knees at the same level as your toes. Also, don't arch or round your back. To push up, you can use your quadriceps, glutes and hamstrings.

Hip Extensions

The hamstrings are probably the most important muscles in your legs. They are not visible, but that doesn't mean they should be ignored. You should treat them the same way as any other muscle in your body. One of the most common exercises to strengthen the hamstrings is hip extensions

Place your back flat on the ground.

Keep your feet flat while you bend your knees.

Lift your hips by squeezing your glutes.

Keep your hand on the ground for a second, then slowly lower down until you hover just above the floor but are not touching it.

To make it more difficult, bend only at the knee. The other leg should be straight and lifted off the ground when lifting.

Forward Lunge

If you do your lunges correctly, they are a great exercise and can be very effective.

Standing at shoulder width, place your feet on the ground.

If you are able, move forward with your right foot.

Keep your left foot on the ground, and bend your right leg towards the ground. Make sure your left knee is bent.

Your right thigh should be parallel to the floor. You don't want to push your knees beyond your toes.

Your upper body should not be bent. Keep your back straight and your hips aligned.

Push your right heel forward to get back up and standing.

Do a set on one side, then switch sides or do alternate sides. Do not step forwards or backwards, but forwards and down.

Walking Lunge

The forward lunge is the easiest way to master. Instead of moving your right leg backwards in the beginning position by extending your right leg forward, keep your left leg straight and move your left leg forward like you were making giant strides in a lunging motion.

Reverse Lunge

You don't have to lunge backwards, but who says that? Start by stepping backwards using one leg. Then, lower your body to the ground and do a forward lunge. The same rules apply: keep your front knee from reaching your toes, bend your back knee towards the ground, and keep your back straight. Keep your stomach in and your spine straight.

Cardiovascular Exercises

Cardiovascular exercise is a must in any exercise program, even one that is focused on fat loss. This type of exercise is what gets your heart pumping and pushes your limits.

Jumping Jacks

This is one of the oldest forms, but it's still one of my favorite exercises. It's great for cardio and warm up.

Keep your arms straight and your shoulders up.

Jump and push your feet to the side. Lift your arms above your head.

Revert to a standing position

Always keep your feet on the ground

Burpees

Burpees, whether you love them or not, are another great form of cardiovascular exercise.

Start form a standing positon

You should lower yourself so your knees are bent, and your hands are flat on the floor.

Straighten your legs so you can push-up.

Get back into a crouch position and get up

Jumping is a great way to get more exercise.

Step-up

These exercises are great for your cardiovascular system and lower body.

A step or strong box should be at least 6 inches tall

Place your right foot in front of the object and stand up.

Push through and squeeze your glutes to lift the left foot up.

Keep it there for a second, then lower it again

Continue to alternate between the left and right sides.

When you feel that this is easy, increase the step but don't go too far.

Mountain Climbers

This is a great exercise to work all your muscles - abs and lower body, as well as your heart.

Start in a push-up position. Make sure your shoulders and hands are aligned.

Bring your abs in, then pull your right leg in towards your chest. The trick is to keep your head straight from head to foot and not tap your toes when your knee touches the ground.

Return your left leg to the beginning and continue with the opposite leg

This will increase your heart rate and speed, and you'll be able to go faster.

Core Exercises

Although you can lose fat however much you want, if your core muscles are not working properly, you'll end up with a flabby stomach. Exercises for the abdominal muscles should be included in any fitness or exercise program.

Plank

Place your back on the ground, face down. Now lift your arms up to your sides. Your shoulders should be parallel to your elbows. Keep your back straight. Keep your feet on the ground.

You can hold this position as long as it is comfortable and then you can lower yourself down.

Side Plank

You can use the same principle as the plank, but this time you will lie on your side, propped on one arm. Hold your hips up and contract your abs. Switch sides by lowering your hips to the ground

Knee up

This exercise will guarantee to get your abs burning.

Grab an overhead bar and hang from it

Bring your knees up to your chest.

Keep your back straight and use your abs instead of your hips.

Keep your knees low and move slowly. Otherwise, your body will continue to rock on the bar.

It All Comes Together

After you've learned all the exercises, make sure to incorporate them all into a circuit training program. Take a few seconds to recover your breath and do one exercise each from each group. You should aim to do six to eight circuits per session. You can modify and remix the exercises to keep your motivation high.

To avoid injury, keep your form correct when exercising. You can also modify an exercise if it is not possible to do the original one. Don't forget about your diet. While you can do many fat-burning exercises, if your diet is poor, you will be unable to lose weight. You should not eat for energy, but the right foods.

Chapter 15: Top Daily Exercises

Benefits

Exercise can be defined as any movement that puts your muscles to work and requires calories to burn.

There are many types of physical activity, including swimming, running, walking, and dancing.

There are many health benefits to being healthy, both mentally and physically. This can help you live longer.

Here are the top ten benefits of daily exercise for the brain and body.

1. You will feel more at ease.

It has been shown that exercise can improve your mood and decrease anxiety.

It can cause brain changes that control anxiety and stress. It can also increase brain responsiveness to the hormones norepinephrine and serotonin, which may help alleviate depression.

Exercise can also increase endorphin production, which is known for its ability to create positive emotions and decrease pain perception.

Anxiety-stricken people can be helped by exercise.

They may also be able to become more aware of their mental health and get rid of their fears.

Surprisingly, it doesn't really matter how intense your workout. No matter how intense the exercise, it seems that the workout will improve your mood.

However, 24 depressed women were found to have significantly lower levels of depression after exercising their strength.

Exercise has such strong mood effects that it is possible to choose to exercise or not for short periods of time.

26 active people were asked by a research team whether they wanted to continue working out for 2 weeks or not. People who quit exercising reported a decrease in their mood.

Regular exercise can boost mood, reduce anxiety, and help with depression.

It will help with weight loss

Numerous studies have shown that obesity and weight gain can be linked to inactivity.

To understand the effect of exercise on weight loss, it is important to understand how energy expenditure and exercise are connected.

The body can expend energy in three ways: by digesting food, exercising, and maintaining bodily functions like the pulse and breathing.

Your metabolic rate will slow down if you eat fewer calories during your diet. Daily exercise can improve your metabolism rate and help you lose weight.

Research has also shown that resistance training combined with aerobic exercise can help to lose fat and maintain muscle mass. This is important for weight loss.

It is important to exercise to increase metabolism and burn calories more frequently. Exercise can also help you lose weight and build muscle.

3. This is great for your bones, and your muscles.

Exercise is crucial for building and maintaining healthy bones and muscles.

When combined with adequate protein intake, physical exercise like weight lifting can help promote muscle building.

Exercise stimulates the release of hormones that increase your body's ability to absorb amino acid. This allows them to thrive and reduces their decay.

As we age, muscle mass and function decreases, leading to disability and injury. Regular exercise is important to maintain strength and decrease muscle loss as you age.

Exercise can help you build bone density and prevent osteoporosis later in life.

Ironically, high-impact activities like running or gymnastics, as well as odd-impact sports like soccer and basketball, have been shown to increase bone density more than other non-impact activities such as swimming or cycling.

Exercise helps to keep bones and muscles strong. This could also help to prevent osteoporosis.

4. It will increase your energy levels

For those who are healthy and for those with various medical conditions, exercise can boost energy.

A study found that 36 people with chronic tiredness reported feeling less tired after six weeks of daily exercise.

People with chronic fatigue syndrome (CFS) or other severe conditions can significantly increase their energy levels by exercising.

CFS treatment seems to be more effective than passive therapies like relaxation and stretching, with exercise being the most successful.

People with progressive diseases such as cancer, HIV/AIDS, multiple sclerosis and other chronic conditions like HIV/AIDS have been found to be more energetic if they exercise.

Daily exercise can increase your energy levels. This is true for both chronically exhausted people and those with severe illnesses.

5. This can lower the chance of developing chronic diseases.

Chronic illness is often caused by a lack of physical activity.

Regular exercise is proven to increase insulin sensitivity, cardiovascular health, and body composition. This can help reduce fat and blood pressure.

A lack of exercise, even in the short-term, can cause significant increases in belly fat. This raises your risk of developing type 2 diabetes, early death, and heart disease.

Regular exercise is recommended to reduce abdominal fat and lower the risk of developing these diseases.

Regular exercise is important for maintaining a healthy weight, and reducing the risk of developing chronic diseases.

6. This will increase the skin's protection.

Your skin can be affected by the amount of oxidative stresses in your body.

When the body's antioxidant defenses are not able to completely repair damage caused by free radicals, oxidative stress is what you see. This can cause damage to their internal structures, and skin can become more brittle.

Exercising for too long can cause oxidative damage. However, moderate exercise can increase your body's natural antioxidants, which protect cells.

Exercise can also increase blood flow, induce adaptations in skin cells and help delay the appearance of skin aging.

Regular exercise can help protect skin from toxins and increase blood flow, which can delay the aging process.

7. It will increase your memory and brain health.

Exercise can improve brain function, preserve memory, and allow you to think more clearly. It increases your heart rate, which facilitates blood flow and oxygen supply to your brain. It can also stimulate hormone production, which may increase brain cell growth.

Exercise can also be beneficial for your brain to prevent chronic diseases. This is because these conditions can cause brain damage. Regular exercise is particularly important for seniors as it can help with brain structure and function.

The hippocampus, which is an essential part of the brain for memory and learning, can be increased by exercise. This can help improve the mental ability of older adults.

Exercise has also been shown to reduce brain changes that can lead to schizophrenia and Alzheimer's disease.

Regular exercise improves blood flow to the brain, and memory and brain health. It can help adults maintain their mental health.

8. This will improve your quality of sleep and relaxation.

You will be able to relax and have a better night's sleep if you do daily workouts. The energy loss that happens during exercise can improve the quality of your sleep. The body's temperature rises during exercise, which is believed to improve the quality of sleep by allowing it fall during sleep. Similar findings have been drawn from many studies on the effects of exercise on sleep.

A study showed that moderate to vigorous activity for 150 minutes per week could increase the quality of sleep by as much as 65%.

Another study found that 17 people with insomnia slept longer and deeper when they did physical exercise for 16 weeks. They also felt more energetic throughout the day.

For those who suffer from sleep disorders, however, it seems that daily exercise is beneficial for them.

Flexibility is key to your choice of exercise. Aerobic exercise, combined with resistance training, can improve your sleep quality. You will feel more energetic and sleep better if you do daily physical activity, whether it's aerobic or resistance training.

9. This will ease your pain

Exercise can reduce chronic pain. Chronic pain can get worse. Chronic pain can be treated with rest and inactivity over a period of time. Recent research shows that exercise can help reduce chronic pain. Multiple studies have shown that exercise can help chronic pain patients reduce their discomfort and improve their quality-of-life.

Numerous studies have shown that exercise can reduce pain from multiple health conditions, such as chronic low back pain, chronic shoulder pain, and chronic soft tissue injury in your shoulder.

Physical exercise can also help to reduce pain perception and pain tolerance.

Exercise can reduce pain related to many conditions. It can also increase your tolerance to pain.

10. It can help you live a more satisfying sex life

Exercising has been shown to increase sex drive

Physical exercise can improve your cardiovascular system, blood circulation, muscle tone, and flexibility. This can all help to enhance your sex life.

Increased physical activity can improve sexual function, sexual satisfaction, as well as increase the frequency of sexual activity

An analysis of 40-year-old women found that they feel more sexual pleasure when they incorporate more intense exercise, such as weight training, sprints and boot camps, into their lives.

A sample of 178 men in good health was examined and found that those who exercised more per week had higher scores for sexual function.

A study found that 41 men experienced erectile dysfunction symptoms by taking a six-minute walk around their house.

Another study of 78 sedentary men found that walking 60 minutes per day (on average three days a week), improved their sexual behaviour. This included duration and satisfaction.

Research has shown that polycystic-ovarian syndrome (which can decrease sex drive) can be improved by daily resistance training.

Women and men can exercise to increase their sexual appetite, work efficiency and productivity. It may also reduce the likelihood of men getting erectile dysfunction.

Exercising can have amazing effects on your health and wellbeing.

Regular exercise can boost hormone output, which makes you happier and allows you to sleep better.

It can improve the appearance of your skin, aid in weight loss, and even help with sex.

You'll see a significant improvement in your health if you do one sport or follow the 150-minute exercise plan per week.

Chapter 16: Simple Lower Abs Workouts for Women at Home

Let me start by saying that humans aren't different in terms of physiology.

Contrasts in the sexual organs are obvious. People are basically the same in all aspects. While we may have different tendencies and inclinations, our bodies are virtually the same.

However, it is a fact that many believe that women should be treated differently to men. I have no idea where it all began, but I do know that it is a side effect of chauvinist culture and thinking we all have from a previous time. This isn't the end of the boring ages! This is why I want to share it with you so that others can perform similar exercises in a similar way.

It is wrong to assume that women can't lift weights and do weight preparation. It is also wrong to assume that women should only do cardio and neglect quality preparing. Women can lift as much as men. Look for female weightlifters who are skilled. They are able to quickly dish it out to men in equal measure!

Most women avoid weight preparation because they fear that they will look too strong and manly. Also, most people don't like strong women. You don't need to worry about getting too strong if you are a woman. Your body doesn't produce enough testosterone to allow you to build muscle mass. Even though people have intense memories of trying to build huge muscles, it's not impossible. It is impossible to get large muscles by weight training.

You'll look more attractive and toned. To achieve their looks, female jocks use a lot of steroids. To look as good as they do, you need to use a lot of enhancements. However, the goal is to look good and be healthy. Basically, ladies can do the same exercises as men and not look like jocks.

Running is the easiest way to get started with working out for women. Running is a great exercise to build lean abs. Many people don't realize that running involves all of the muscles, including the abs. They should start their exercise program with running. Runs are the best way to start running.

You should be energetic. If you could in a sense run for your lives because you were being chased by wild animals, that would be the best kind of power you should have when you run.

Your diet is the next thing you should focus on to shape your abs. These are the most important principles. First, avoid grains. Second, avoid sugar in all its forms (counting natural product squeeze). Third, keep a strategic distance away from any handled food or beverages. Fourth, stay away from hydrogenated oils. Fifth, avoid bland vegetables. It is also important to eat leafy vegetables with caution.

For abdominal muscle exercise, the next thing is to get sufficient sleep in the evening and enough daylight throughout the day. Because of the many benefits you receive from getting enough rest and daylight, your body's ability to see the world from different perspectives is important.

Simple but effective home workouts for women

Every woman in the world dreams of a slim and fit body. Many women these days are unable to afford an exercise center membership or don't have the time or money to go to the rec center. If you are one of these women, you need to search for the best way to exercise at home for ladies.

These are some simple tips:

If your home has a step, you can walk up it and then descend. This is a great way to get your workouts started. If you are able to fit in a few more steps per day, that is even better.

Use the divider to divide your space and do some push-ups. Keep your hands as far away from the divider as possible. Continue to place your hands on the divider's upper side and then spread them out at any point you do push-ups.

Adjustment practices can be done by balancing on one foot and putting your other foot on the front or back. For women, adjusting practices can be a great exercise to do at home. They could help you strengthen your center leg muscles. This is why you should do it as often as possible.

A clothing bag that is full of garments can be used for arm chiseling. The container can be placed on your head, and you can then lift it up. Do three repetitions of this exercise. If the container is too heavy to carry, you can take the garments out.

Take some large jars of food from your pantry and put them together. Use the jars to lose weight and do all of the free weight exercises you can. If you own a very heavy can, try to raise it twofold. Use a seat with wheels. A turn seat is an excellent choice. You can do arm exercises before you go to work by holding onto the edge of your work space while still sitting on your seat. Use your arm muscles to move closer to the work area and then slowly drive away.

If you have a large foyer in your home or a section that has a long passageway, then this area can be used to perform knee twists. You can finish this by walking along the walkway with your knees, starting at one end and moving to the next. You can also try to walk down the walkway in all fours or do line moves or a reverse crab walk.

Play a bicycle on the ground, laying flat on your back. You can even use your feet to cut. You should make sure your floors are clean before you start.

Conclusion

Next, you need to create space in your home for home exercise. Consider what household equipment you will use. Get your sticky notes ready. It's time to stop wishing and get a better body.

You can meal prep on Sundays, or any other night that works for you. This is a simple step that will simplify your life. This will help you get enough results. Be creative! You will be grateful that you have more time.

Get motivated to do your workouts by investing in a whiteboard. This book is designed to help you build a strong, healthy body. We want to help you make the most of all that you have learned and show you what you can do. You won't know until you actually try.

Only one life and only one body are available to you. Do not let yourself be swayed by laziness or slothfulness. Be courageous. Be strong. You have the world at your disposal. All the best.

www.ingramcontent.com/pod-product-compliance
Lightning Source LLC
Chambersburg PA
CBHW062224020426
42397CB00018B/150